Zone Diet

Explore Efficient And Uncomplicated Recipes That Are Abundant In Essential Nutrients, Along With Well-Established Customs And Nourishing Practices That Promote Longevity And Vibrant Well-Being

(An Architectural Plan For A Lively And Prolonged Existence)

HanspeterDraxler

TABLE OF CONTENT

Blue Zone Foods 1

Tacos With Sweet Potatoes And Black Beans 4

Clutches About Prevention On The Blue Zones Diet 27

Blue Zones' Red Lentil Soup 34

Blue Zone Food Recommendations 36

Sautéed Zucchini Parm 50

Occasional Egg 54

Japanese Miso Soup: Savoury Drink For Extended Lifespan 82

Blue Zone Dietary Guidelines 84

Veggie Breakfast Burritos 96

Greek Salad 102

Apple Cinnamon Quinoa 104

Recipes For Blue Zone Green Smoothies 105

Blue Zone Foods

The Blue Zone Diet is a nutritional approach that has become well-known because it is associated with the longevity of those residing in "Blue Zones," where people often live longer, healthier lives—often exceeding 100 years of age.

All Blue Zone communities have a common diet, which emphasizes particular foods and eating habits that add to their extraordinary lifespan. Here, we examine the key elements of the Blue Zone Diet:

Produce and Fruits

The core of the Blue Zone Diet is an abundance of fruits and vegetables. These plant-based dishes contain fiber, vitamins, minerals, and antioxidants. They are vital in improving overall health and reducing the risk of chronic disorders. Their diet residents of the Blue Zones consume various vibrant vegetables, leafy greens, and seasonal fruits.

Complete Grains

In Blue Zone communities, you may often get. These grains are rich in fiber, other minerals, and complex carbohydrates, which lowers the risk of heart disease and diabetes.

Legumes

Residents of the Blue Zone frequently consume legumes, including chickpeas, lentils, and beans. These legumes are rich in essential minerals, fiber, and plant-based protein. Satiety, and help maintain a healthy weight.

Seeds and Nuts

The Blue Zone Diet includes a lot of nuts and seeds. Nuts like walnuts, flaxseeds, and almonds are frequently included. These meals offer various health benefits, including a.

Fish

In regions where there is access to the Blue Zone Diet. Because of their heart- and brain-healthy properties, omega-3 fatty acids make fatty fish—like salmon and mackerel—very popular. Consuming seafood is associated with a lower risk of cardiovascular disease in people living in the Blue Zone.

Lacto-fermented Foods

There are certain Blue Zone regions where dairy consumption is moderate. Yogurt and cheese are two common meals. Probiotics included in fermented foods like sauerkraut and kimchi are also highly valued since they improve overall health and intestinal health.

Spices and Herbs

People in the Blue Zone season their cuisine with herbs and spices instead of using a lot of sugar or salt. Spices like cinnamon, turmeric and herbs like oregano and rosemary provide several health benefits, from improved digestion to anti-inflammatory properties.

Besides the designated meals, the Blue Zone Diet is characterized by mindful eating practices. Blue Zone cuisine emphasizes sharing meals with others, eating till full, and using smaller portions. These actions enhance overall well-being and add to the remarkably long lifespans of those residing there.

Ultimately, the Blue Zone Diet offers a pattern for a long and healthy life by emphasizing plant-based foods, whole grains, legumes, nuts, seafood, and a balanced approach to dairy and fermented foods. This approach shows how nutrition can improve overall health and lifespan when paired with mindful eating practices. Whether one follows the Blue Zone Diet's exact food list or just adopts its principles, incorporating these elements into one's diet may result in a more contented and energetic life.

Tacos With Sweet Potatoes And Black Beans

Ingredients:
- 1 can black beans, rinsed and drained
- 1/2 cup diced tomatoes

- 1/4 cup chopped cilantro
- **2 sweet potatoes, peeled and diced**
- 1 tablespoon olive oil
- 1 teaspoon chili powder
- 1/2 teaspoon ground cumin
- 1/2 teaspoon paprika
- Salt and pepper to taste
- Corn tortillas
- **Optional toppings:** avocado slices, salsa, shredded lettuce

Instructions:

1. Sweet potatoes should be nicely coated after being tossed in a bowl with olive oil,
2. Chilli powder, cumin, paprika, salt, and pepper.
3. After spreading out on a baking sheet, bake the seasoned sweet potatoes for 20 to 25

minutes or until they are soft and starting to color.
4. Add chopped cilantro, diced tomatoes, and black beans to a small bowl.
5. Place corn tortillas on a dry skillet and heat it to medium.
6. Spoon the black bean mixture and roasted sweet potatoes into each tortilla.
7. If desired, add the optional toppings.
8. Warm up and serve.

MANAGING A HEALTHY DIET THAT WORKS FOR YOU

One of the numerous components of daily existence is food.

Food could be the last thing on your mind after work, errands, family or social obligations, and commuting, among other everyday concerns.

Making food a priority is the first step in eating a better diet.

Spending hours cooking elaborate dinners or preparing meals is unnecessary, but it does need some planning and work, particularly if you lead a hectic lifestyle.

I suggest sensible and successful diets like the Zone, maybe in a Mediterranean variant.

WHAT Eating in the Zone entails

THE ZONE'S FUNDAMENTAL TENES

Despite what some individuals believe, the Zone diet has clear and easy principles.

Then, in certain situations, we might argue that it is just common sense.

The well-known 40/30/30 quantitative rule solves the issue of calculating the calories of individual foods.

It is imperative that 40% of the calories we consume come from carbohydrates, 30% from proteins, and 30% from fats.

Simple tables make this possible.

PARTITIONING OUT MEALS

Meals must be spread out across a full day. Specifically, there should be no more than 4/5 hours between a main meal and a snack and no more than 3 hours between a snack and the next meal (not including nights).

Having a snack 30 minutes before bed is best.

This also depends on our schedules, but trying to come as close as possible is still helpful, even if it isn't always feasible.

This is eating before you are truly hungry, which frequently results in overindulging in food and consuming the incorrect kinds of food.

THE FOOD QUALITY

The Zone diet strongly emphasizes dietary quality.

Thus, it is especially advised to utilize wholegrain grasses as a secondary source of carbs and to use fruits and vegetables as the primary source.

Utilizing mono and polyunsaturated fats—found in olive oil, dried fruit, and the fat of some fish, such as oily fish—is advised by the Zone diet.

Since the Omega 3 series fats are so important, special attention is paid to them.

Lean proteins are desired, focusing on fish and white meat in particular. Vegetable proteins, like those found in legumes, should never be completely absent.

Thus, in general, the Zone diet aligns with the Mediterranean diet, which I discussed right after, at least regarding food quality.

NOT ONLY FOOD

The Zone diet strongly emphasizes physical exercise as a vital component of lifestyle—not just for those who need to lose weight but also for those of normal weight. This is something I think is important.

Our bodies could never function to their fullest capacity, even with a proper, balanced diet like the Zone, if we did not engage in intellectual, deliberate physical activity. I am referring to physical exercise here, not sport, as the latter is more often than not competitive and so a cause of stress as opposed to wellbeing.

Since learning about the Zone diet, I have also been drawn to its emphasis on using relaxation or meditation techniques as a stress-reduction strategy.

Ignoring stress can render our attention to food and physical activity pointless, as it has a significant impact not only on our weight and physical appearance but also on our overall health.

2.1 Comprehending the Blue Zone Way of Life

Understanding the more holistic way of life that contributes to the remarkable health of Blue Zone residents is crucial to appreciating the Blue Zone diet and its effects on longevity. Their extraordinary longevity is partly attributed to their way of life, relationships, and sense of purpose rather than the food on their plates.

2.1.1 Robust Social Networks

Blue Zone communities' strong sense of social connectivity is one of their defining characteristics. They cultivate strong, long-lasting bonds with neighbors, family, and friends. These social ties improve general wellbeing by lowering stress, fostering a sense of belonging, and offering emotional support.

2.1.1.1 Families with Multiple Generations

Living alongside one another or in close contact throughout generations regularly occurs in several Blue Zones. Living with different generations together makes the elderly feel more connected to one another, gives them a purpose in life, and keeps them engaged in day-to-day activities.

2.1.2 Vigorous Ways of Living

The daily habits of those living in the Blue Zone incorporate physical activity. They walk, garden, and perform manual labor as regular, moderate-intensity physical activity. These exercises improve muscular strength, flexibility, and cardiovascular health.

2.1.2.1 Organic Motion*

Natural mobility is a common part of Blue Zone populations' daily life. This includes walking to see neighbors, gardening, and participating in dance performances during community events. These pleasurable and long-lasting exercise styles improve general fitness.

2.1.3 Techniques for Relaxation and Stress Reduction

One essential component of the Blue Zone lifestyle is stress management. Residents prioritize unwinding and reducing stress by engaging in activities like meditation, prayer, or just spending time with loved ones. These methods lessen the damaging impact that long-term stress has on one's health.

2.1.4 A Feeling of Intent

People who live in the Blue Zone frequently have a strong feeling of purpose from their community involvement. Having a purpose in life, whether it is taking care of grandchildren, maintaining local customs, or mentoring the next generation, is linked to better mental and emotional health.

2.1.5 Recuperation and Rest Period

It is impossible to overestimate the value of relaxation and sound sleep in today's busy world. People living in the Blue Zone place a high value on getting enough sleep; they frequently nap every day and stick to regular sleep regimens. A good night's sleep is essential to their general health.

As we delve into the culinary components of these exceptional places, it is imperative to comprehend the comprehensive nature of the Blue Zone lifestyle. It serves as a reminder that the Blue Zone diet is only one component of the jigsaw; social interactions, physical activity, emotional stability, and proper nutrition all work together harmoniously to give these people long and healthy lives.

According to research, strong social ties and lower stress levels include longer life expectancy. A 2010 study that appeared to have a 50% higher chance of survival was linked to social integration.

2.2 The Longevity Science

The Blue Zone diet is a scientifically based strategy for improving health and prolonging human life, not merely a collection of dietary customs handed down through the years. Experts and researchers have examined Blue Zone populations in great detail, revealing the fundamental science behind their way of life's remarkable longevity-promoting effects.

2.2.1 Nutrition's Function

The food habits of the Blue Zone are a major factor in their lifespan. Numerous essential components of the Blue Zone diet that support lifespan and good health have been discovered by researchers:

2.2.1.1 Foods High in Antioxidants

Antioxidant-rich foods abound in blue zone diets. These substances, abundant in fruits and vegetables, fight aging and chronic illnesses.

2.2.1.2 Good Fats for the Heart

Cardiovascular health is supported by consuming heart-healthy fats, especially nuts and olive oil. These fats assist in lowering the risk of heart disease, which is one of the world's leading causes of death.

2.2.1.3 Macronutrients in Balance

A balanced macronutrient ratio is typical of blue zone diets, which focus on complex carbs, moderate protein intake, and low saturated fat. This equilibrium supports stable blood sugar levels and general health.

Numerous studies on animals have demonstrated that calorie restriction increases lifespan and enhances metabolic health. Although research on humans is still in progress, data from animal studies points to a possible influence on longevity1.

2.2.2 The Effects of Eating Plant-Based Diets

The health advantages of plant-based diets, such as those seen in the Blue Zones, have been well-researched. The following is the science underlying longevity and plant-based diets:

2.2.2.1 Reduced Chronic Illness Rates

Diets high in plants are linked to heart disease and several types of cancer. Diets in the Blue Zones are rich in plant foods, which helps explain why disease prevalence is lower there.

2.2.2.2 Better Digestive Health

Plant-based diets' high fiber content helps to maintain. Better general health and a more robust immune system are associated with healthy gut flora.

2.2.3 The Impact of the Mediterranean

Longevity in Blue Zones like Sardinia and Ikaria is largely attributed to the Mediterranean diet. Among the scientific foundations of the Mediterranean diet are:

2.2.3.1 Advantages of Cardiovascular

The Mediterranean diet offers a beneficial dietary balance that lowers the risk of heart disease and stroke because it strongly emphasizes whole grains, fish, and olive oil.

2.2.3.2 Mental Wellbeing

According to research, a Mediterranean diet may help guard against neurological illnesses, including Alzheimer's and age-related cognitive decline.

2.2.4 The Lifestyle's Effect

The science of longevity in Blue Zones includes lifestyle aspects in addition to diet:

2.2.4.1 Extended Lifespan and Social Networks

Blue Zones, encouraging social engagement and lowering stress levels. It is believed that eating in groups enhances wellbeing in general.

According to research, strong social ties and lower stress levels include longer life expectancy. A 2010 study that appeared to have a 50% higher chance of survival was linked to social integration.

2.2.4.2 Vitality and Physical Activity

Frequent physical activity promotes cardiovascular health, muscular strength, and general vitality, even in mild, daily activities like walking.

Comprehending the scientific basis for the longevity of the Blue Zone highlights the significance of embracing their food and lifestyle practices. It's not just anecdotal; several scientific studies have confirmed it. You're making decisions that could greatly impact your lifetime and health by adopting the Blue Zone way of life.

2.3 The Benefits of a Plant-Based Diet

the Lifespan and Vigorous of Blue Zone Residents.

It will help you make informed dietary decisions.

The advantages of plant-based diets for health are regularly demonstrated by scientific research. As an illustration, a 2019 that follows a (CHD)2.

2.3.1 Nutrient Abundance

Diets based primarily on plants are high in key elements important for general health. Communities in the Blue Zone consume a broad range of plant foods, such as:

2.3.1.1 Vibrant Greens

Various vibrant veggies offer an array of vitamins, minerals, and antioxidants. These nutrients lessen inflammation, boost the immune system, and guard against long-term illnesses.

2.3.1.2 Fruits High in Nutrients

Fruits are a natural source of natural sugars, fiber, and vitamins. They have several advantages, including boosting heart health, improving digestion, and supplying vital antioxidants.

Plant Proteins 2.3.1.3

excellent providers of plant-based protein. They also include a lot of fiber, promoting digestion and fullness.

2.3.1.4 Complete Cereals

Nutrient-dense whole grains include quinoa, brown rice, and oats. Fibre and long-lasting energy.

2.3.2 Longevity and Heart Health

Among the advantages are:

Reduced Levels of Cholesterol-lowering LDL cholesterol.

2.3.2.2 Control of Blood Pressure

Healthy blood pressure is facilitated by a plant-based diet's abundance of fruits and vegetables that are high in potassium.

2.3.2.3 Lower Chance of Chronic Illnesses

Diets based primarily on plants are linked to a decreased risk of developing chronic illnesses.

2.3.3 Controlling Your Weight

Plant-based diets are useful for managing weight since they frequently include fewer calories per serving.

2.3.4 Immunity and Gut Health

Plant-based diets contain fiber, which helps maintain a balanced gut microbiota. Inflammation and improved immunity are linked to a diversified and well-balanced gut microbiota.

2.3.5 Sustainability of the Environment

Eating a plant-based diet has been shown to have a positive environmental impact.

Adopting the Blue Zone diet's tenets requires first realizing the benefits of a plant-based diet. You can take advantage of the nutritional advantages that lead to longer life, greater health, and a more sustainable future by increasing the amount of plant-based foods in your diet.

Plant-centric Blue Zone recipes in the upcoming chapters highlight the delectable tastes and wellbeing advantages of plant-centric cooking.

Knowing About Carbs on the Zone Diet

The Zone Diet heavily relies on carbohydrates as a source of energy, fiber, and other nutrients. On the other hand, the Zone Diet emphasizes using low-GI carbohydrates to support overall metabolic balance and sustain stable blood sugar levels. The following are some essential elements of comprehending carbs in the Zone Diet:

Glycemic index: Carbohydrates are ranked according to how they affect blood sugar levels using the glycemic index (GI). A key component of the Zone Diet is ingesting low-glycemic carbs. Because these carbohydrates take longer to break down and absorb, the blood gradually releases glucose into the bloodstream. This promotes improved glycemic management and lessens the risk of blood sugar rises.

Fiber content: The Zone Diet encourages eating a lot of high-fiber carbs. Improved satiety, better blood sugar regulation, and better digestion are just a few of the health advantages of fiber. To boost fiber intake and advance general health, include carbohydrates high in fiber in your meals.

Portion control is crucial, even if the Zone Diet requires many carbohydrates. In the Zone Diet, 40% of each meal is usually made up of carbohydrates. You can sustain stable blood sugar levels and a balanced intake of macronutrients by controlling portion sizes and making intelligent carbohydrate choices.

Entire, unprocessed carbohydrates: Eating entire, unprocessed carbohydrates is emphasized in the Zone Diet. Phytochemicals and whole carbs tend to be higher than refined or processed carbohydrates. They contribute to total food intake and offer sustained energy.

Individualized needs for carbohydrates: The Zone Diet acknowledges that a person's needs for carbohydrates may differ depending on several variables, including activity level, desired body composition, and metabolic response. It's crucial to customize your carbohydrate consumption to meet your unique needs. For advice about your objectives, speak with a qualified dietitian or other healthcare provider.

Balanced macronutrient distribution: The Zone Diet encourages balanced macronutrient distribution, with 40% of each meal from carbs. This equilibrium, combined with sufficient protein and good fats, aids in sustaining steady insulin levels, regulating appetite, and promoting metabolic balance.

When adding carbohydrates to your Zone Diet, go for whole, unprocessed foods high in fiber and low on the glycemic index. Add vibrant fruits and vegetables, nutritious grains like brown rice or quinoa, and legumes like chickpeas or lentils.

Remember that everyone has a varied tolerance for carbohydrates, so it's critical to watch how your body reacts to various kinds and quantities of food. Adapt your carbohydrate intake to your unique needs, objectives, and any dietary restrictions you may have.

Engaging with a trained dietitian can offer tailored direction and assistance in comprehending and controlling carbs within the framework of the Zone Diet. Optimally nutritionally adequate and in line with your goals.

Clutches About Prevention On The Blue Zones Diet

Everyone has been taught that protein is necessary to develop strong bones and muscles in our bodies, but how much is the right amount? The typical American woman consumes 70 grams of protein daily, but the average man consumes more than 100 grams: Way too much. It is 46 to 56 grams per day. However, quantity doesn't matter. We also require the appropriate type of prevention. Pite—referred to as amino acids—occurs in 21 different forms. The body cannot produce any known as the. All-natural amino acids are found in meat and eggs, but few plant food sources do. However, meat and eggs also include fat and cholesterol, which tend to worsen heart disease and cancer. How, then, do you go about following the Blue Zones diet and emphasizing plant-based foods? The secret is to "pair" specific foods with each other. Combining the appropriate plant sources. You will satisfy your protein requirements and monitor your caloric consumption.

Recipe made with meat

Eat meat no more frequently than twice a week. Eat meals twice a week, or even less frequently, if you're satisfied with no more than two cooked ounces. Choose genuine free-range chicken and lamb from family-farmed farms over meats bred in industrial settings. Clear processed foods like hot dogs, luncheon meats, and sausages.

Most Blue Zone diets consist of small poultry, chicken, or lamb portions. (The exception being Adventists, who consumed no meat at all.) Families traditionally cook their pigs or goats for festivals, feasts, and funerals. The leftovers would then be used, sometimes as flavoring and sometimes as fat for frying. Chickens roamed the land, eating grasshoppers and building their roosts. However, like rare meats, chicken meat was enjoyed sparingly over various meals.

By averaging meat consumption across all Blue Zones, we discovered that individuals consumed small amounts of meat, approximately two or fewer servings at a time, five times a month. They were stolen about once a month, generally from a roasted goat or pig. Neither beef nor Turkish fries significantly contribute to the average Blue Zone diet.

Free-Range Meats

The best individuals in the Blue Zones work as free-roaming animations. These animals do not suffer from the symptoms of large fevers since they are not dosed with hormones, phenolphthaleinoids, or antibiotics. Goats continuously feed on grass, foliage, and twigs. Pigs from Sardinia and Ikaria eat chicken scraps and use them as fuel for their woven tents and rugs. The meat from these conventionally raised animals, probably.

Furthermore, we don't know if people lived longer in the Blue Zones because they ate a small amount of meat or if they survived despite it. Since there are so many healthy practices that Blue Zone members engage in, it's possible that they were able to get past eating a small amount of meat because other food and lifestyle choices counterbalanced its harmful effects. As my buddy Dan Ornish said, "The more healthy practices you adopt, the healthier you become."

How to go about doing it:

Find out what two ounces of cooked meat looks like. Chicken: around half a breast fillet or the meat (not the skin) of a chicken leg. Before cooking, chop or slice a pork or lamb the size of a deck.

Steer clear of bringing beef, hot dogs, luncheon meats, poultry, or other processed meats into your home, as they are not included in the Blue Zones diet.

Discover plant-based substitutes for the supper that Americans are accustomed to having at the end of a meal. Try gently salted tofu drizzled with olive oil, tempeh, another soy product, plain bread, or chocolate chip cakes.

Choose to consume meat or other animal-derived foods twice a week and limit your enjoyment to those days.

Given that restaurant portion sizes are often four ounces or more, split the meal with another person or allow a customer to take half of the meal portion home for later.

Continue to Move

People in these areas are rarely seen throughout the day. Some people live in extremely difficult environments, such as hills, where walking is their primary mode of transportation and exercise is an integral part of their daily routine rather than the gym. They are constantly on their feet.

Move more, even if your work requires you to sit down most of the day. When it's closer to work, walk there instead of taking a taxi. Take your papers from the next office and brew coffee rather than order one.

Use these tactics to complete a 10,000-step walk while working a desk job.

Consume More Blue Zone Foods

In addition to beans, other foods included in the Blue Zones diet include nuts, sweet potatoes, cauliflower, apples, pears, leafy greens, and turmeric.

Replace your cooking olive oil with the healthier kind, which you can use not only for cooking but also to dress salads and bake with.

Consume Wine Cautionfully

Prominent features were observed in the diets that underwent analysis. For example, in the Sardinia region of Italy, the people ascribed their long life to the locally produced wine made from Grenache grapes.

Take note, though—most of the wine consumed was produced locally.

Second, the wine was used sparingly, usually following a day of physically demanding activities. This does not mean you should have a bottle of red wine every morning!

Drinks Without Sweeteners

They had unsweetened black coffee as they were drinking it. If they used any honey at all, it was natural honey.

To follow this diet, prepare raw vegetables, candied fruits, and other processed foods indoors. Ensure not to use excessive honey, which would defeat the objective of cutting out sugar.

Eat most of your daily fruit from fruits, much like the adventures.

Having Breakfast Like A King

You know their customs: breakfast like a king, dinner like a pauper. This phrase rings true for most of the Blue Zones' diet.

The most prominent food groups are found in the first meal, which is HUGE. The day's final meal is often small and consumed either very early in the evening or late in the afternoon. Evenings are meant for rest.

Blue Zones' Red Lentil Soup

Ingredients:

- 1 bagof red lentils (16 oz)
- 1 ¼ teaspoonturmeric
- ½ teaspoon cumin
- 10 cups of water
- Saltandpeppertoseason
- 1 tablespoonoliveoil
- 1 medium onion, diced
- 3 cloves garlic, chopped
- 5 stalksofcelery, diced

Instructions

1. Heat oil in a big pot with 4 to 5 quarts over medium heat until heated but not cooked.
2. After that, cook for about two minutes or until golden.
3. For one to two minutes, stir in celery, turmeric, cumin, ginger, and sauté.
4. Pour in the water and heat until it boils. Simmer, stirring occasionally.
5. Until the lentils become tender, about 20 minutes. Season to taste with pepper and salt.
6. This is a really simple recipe made with basic ingredients. However, you might add ingredients like carrots, parsley, or cilantro.
7. In case you don't have turmeric or cumin, you can use curry seasoning as a substitute.
8. Use one can of unsweetened coconut instead.

Blue Zone Food Recommendations

If you adhere to these guidelines, you will eat more whole, nutrient-dense, and fiber-rich foods—all in a naturally occurring manner.

Plant Angle

Ninety-five percent of your food is derived from plants or plant products. To no more than one small dish each day. Favorite vegetables: potatoes, carrots, squash, nuts, and seeds. Whole grains are also okay. Even though people consume meat in four of the five Blue Zones, they do it differently. Some use it as a side dish, a celebration food, or a way to flavor vegetables. As our advisor Walter Willett of the Harvard School of Public Health put it: "We don't know the safe level of meat."

Furthermore, research indicates that 30-year-old vegetarian Adventists are likely to outlive their meat-eating companions by as much as several years. Numerous health benefits.

When in season, inhabitants in the Blue Zones consume a wide variety of garden vegetables, which they subsequently pickle or dry to enjoy during the off-season. The best long-lasting foods in the Blue Zones diet include leafy greens, spinach, collards, beet and turnip tops, carrots, and cilantro. More than 75 different types of edible plants grow like weeds in Indonesia; the phytosterols in red wine are frequently found in weeds. Research has shown that middle-aged individuals who consumed the equivalent of half a cup of cooked green beans every day were half as likely to die in the next four years as those who did not eat any green beans. Additionally, researchers discovered that individuals who consumed a quarter of a pound of fruit daily (about an ounce) had a 60% lower chance of dying during the next four years than those who did not. Many oils come from plants and are all preferred to animal-based fats. Although we cannot claim that olive oil is the only healthy plant-based oil, it is the most frequently utilized in the Blue Zone diet. There is proof that a low-fat diet raises good cholesterol and lowers bad cholesterol. In Iceland, we discovered that approximately five tablespoons of olive oil daily appeared to cut the risk of death in half for middle-aged people. Healthy grains and beans take center stage when mixed with seasonal fruits and vegetables. Blue Zones offers year-round meals and snacks.

How to go about doing it:

Always have your favorite fruits and vegetables on hand. Avoid trying to make yourself eat something you don't enjoy. That might function for a while, but it will fizzle out sooner or later. Try a variety of fruits and vegetables; identify which ones you enjoy and keep your kitchen well-stocked with them. Frozen vegetables will do if you don't have access to fresh, reasonably priced vegetables. (In actuality, because they were flash-frozen during harvest rather than traveling for weeks to your local grocery store's shelves, they frequently contain more nutrients.)

Apply olive oil like a butt. Sauté veggies in olive oil over low heat. Additionally, you can finish boiling or steaming vegetables by brushing them with a small amount of extra virgin olive oil, which you should keep on your table.

Glue up the entire grain. We discovered that oatmeal, barley, broccoli, and ground corn were included in Blue Zone diets worldwide. In these cultures, wheat played a minor role, and the grains they utilized contained less gluten than the modern grains of today.

Whatever vegetables are left in your fridge can be turned into vegetable soup by cutting them, browning them with olive oil and herbs, and adding boiling water to cover them. Simmer until the vegetables are tender, and then season to taste. Freeze what you don't have time to cook in individual or family-sized containers, then serve later in the week or month.

Information about Protein in the Blue Zones Diet

Everyone has been taught that protein is necessary to develop strong bones and muscles in our bodies, but how much is the right amount? The typical American woman consumes 70 grams of protein daily, but the average man consumes more than 100 grams: Way too much. It is 46 to 56 grams per day. However, quantity doesn't matter. We also require the appropriate type of prevention. Pite—referred to as amino acids—occurs in 21 different forms. The body cannot produce any known as the. All-natural amino acids are found in meat and eggs, but few plant food sources do. However, meat and eggs also include fat and cholesterol, which tend to worsen heart disease and cancer. How, then, do you go about following the Blue Zones diet and emphasizing plant-based foods? The secret is to "pair" specific foods with each other. Combining the appropriate plant sources. You will satisfy your protein requirements and monitor your caloric consumption.

SWEET POTATO PANCAKES IN OKINAWAN SW

This is a step-by-step guide for making Okinawan Sweet Potato Pancakes simple enough for beginners to follow.

Sweet Potato Pancakes from Okinawa: Sunshine on a Plate

Ingredients: Pure sweet potatoes from Okinawa

A small amount of honey (optional) on eggs

cooking oil

Steps:

Assemble your ingredients:

Begin by gathering all of your ingredients. You will need eggs, Okinawan purple sweet potatoes, some cooking oil, and, if desired, a hint of honey.

Assemble the sweet potatoes:

Peel the sweet potatoes from Okinawa to start. They might need to be peeled similarly to regular potatoes. Rinse them under cold water to get rid of any dirt.

Slice the sweet potatoes:

Cut the sweet potatoes into small pieces after peeling. The pieces will cook more quickly the smaller they are. Try to make cubes that are roughly half an inch in size.

Simmer the Sweet Potatoes:

Put the chopped sweet potatoes into a boiling pot of water. Allow them to cook until they are soft and mushy. This usually takes fifteen to twenty minutes. You may test their doneness by inserting a fork easily into a piece; it should slide in easily.

Funky and drain:

After the sweet potatoes are tender, remove the hot water from the vehicle and allow it to cool for a few minutes. They must be sufficiently chilled for you to handle them easily.

Grind the Sweet Potatoes:

Have a smooth consistency. You may leave little lumps if you prefer a particular texture.

Get the batter ready:

Generally, one egg per cup of mashed sweet potatoes works well, but the amount of eggs you use will depend on how many sweet potatoes you have.

Drizzle some honey into the batter if desired. Suppose you'd like to add sweetness to your baked eggs. Since Okinawan sweet potatoes are sweet, this step is optional.

Blend and blend:

Beaten eggs and honey (if using). Mix everything until you get a homogenous batter. It should be smooth and thick.

Warm up the pan:

Heat a frying pan over medium-high heat by placing it on the stove. Add a small amount of cooking oil and let it warm up.

Get the pancakes ready for dinner.

After the oil has heated up, spoon some sweet potato batter into the pan to form a pancake. They can be made to whatever size you choose.

Swivel and get supper ready:

Allow the cake to cook until you notice bubbles starting to appear on the surface, which usually takes a few minutes. After that, thoroughly flip it over and cook dinner on the other side until it turns golden brown.

Repeat and tolerate the heat:

Repeat the procedure using the remaining battery, adding extra oil to the pan as necessary. Once the baking process is complete, you can keep the cakes warm in an oven set to a low temperature.

Serve and savor:

Now that your Okinawan Sweet Potato Pancakes are prepared, they can be served. They are delicious, but if you want to add even more sweetness, you may drizzle more honey.

Clean Up:

After you've enjoyed your pancakes, clean your kitchen and kitchenware. A thief's best friend is a tidy workspace!

That's it! You've made Okinawan Sweet Potato Pancakes, a distinctive and delightful breakfast inspired by the Okinawan Blue Zone, where these sweet potatoes are prized for their inherent sweetness and health advantages. Savor the splendor of your hometown on a plate!

The Theory of Hormonal Balance

According to hormonal balance, hormones preserve general health and wellbeing. Hormones are chemical messengers that control many biological processes, including growth, metabolism, mood, and reproduction. Different glands in the body produce them. This idea holds that good physical and mental health depends on preserving a delicate hormonal balance.

1. Important Hormones: The intricate regulatory system of the body is influenced by multiple hormones. A few of the important hormones are:

Promoting fertility and fostering the emergence of secondary sexual traits.

The main sex hormone in men, testosterone, affects libido, bone density, muscle mass, and general vigor.

Insulin: The pancreas secretes insulin, which helps cells absorb glucose and controls blood sugar levels.

Cortisol: The adrenal glands release cortisol, which affects immunological response, metabolism, and how the body reacts to stress.

Which control growth, development, and metabolism.

2. Hormonal Imbalances: A disturbance in the delicate hormone balance can result in several health problems. Stress, a poor diet, inactivity, certain medical problems, and aging-related

changes are all potential causes of hormonal imbalances.

Typical Symptoms: A variety of symptoms, such as exhaustion, mood swings, weight gain or loss, irregular menstrual cycles, reduced libido, hair loss, and sleep difficulties, can indicate hormonal imbalances.

Health Implications: Diabetes, infertility, hypo- or hyperthyroidism, polycystic ovarian syndrome (PCOS), and other disorders can all be influenced by hormonal imbalances.

3. Effect on Health: According to the notion of hormonal balance, hormone abnormalities can significantly impact one's general health and wellbeing.

Hormones are mostly responsible for controlling hunger and metabolism and managing weight. These processes can be hampered by hormonal imbalances, resulting in weight gain or making it harder to lose weight.

Mood and Mental Health: Variations in hormone levels, especially in progesterone and estrogen, can affect mood and exacerbate disorders, including postpartum depression and premenstrual syndrome (PMS).

Energy Levels: Disproportions in thyroid hormones, particularly in cortisol, can affect hormone levels. Hypothyroidism, or low thyroid function, can cause weariness and lethargy, whereas prolonged stress, or high cortisol levels, can cause persistent exhaustion.

4. Management and Treatment: Taking care of hormonal abnormalities frequently requires a diversified strategy.

Lifestyle Changes: Hormone balance can be achieved through a balanced diet, stress reduction strategies, and enough sleep.

Hormone Replacement Treatment: In certain situations, hormone replacement treatment may be advised to restore hormonal balance.

This method is frequently applied to diseases, including hypothyroidism and menopause.

Targeted Medications: Certain drugs may be recommended to treat particular hormonal disorders. For instance, hormonal acne and menstrual cycle regulation are two benefits of birth control tablets.

The Ratio of Zones

Dr. Barry Sears created the well-known Zone Ratio eating plan in the 1990s. The main objective is to get a particular balance of macronutrients to enhance hormone response, manage inflammation, and advance general wellbeing. The Zone Ratio, often known as the "40-30-30" ratio, denotes the proportion of calories that need to originate from fat, protein, and carbs in that order. Let's examine the tenets and advantages of this idea in more detail.

Fundamentals of the Zone Ratio

The Zone Ratio's foundation is that the ratio of macronutrients in a meal or diet can affect the body's hormonal response, specifically the synthesis of eicosanoids, glucagon, and insulin. The Zone Ratio seeks to accomplish a number of weight management, decreased inflammation, and sharper mental focus by carefully regulating these hormone reactions.

Sautéed Zucchini Parm

Ingredients

- 6. ½ medium red onion, diced
- 7. ½ cupfresh basil leaves, torn
- 2 cloves garlic, roughlychopped
- 4 ozfreshmozzarella cheese, sliced 1/4-inch thick

- Crushedred pepper flakes, forserving (optional)
- GratedParmesan cheese, for serving (optional)
- Toastedbread or pasta (gluten-free, if
- necessary), for serving (optional)
- 2 lbs (about 3–4 medium) zucchini, halved lengthwise
- 2. 1/4 cupoliveoil
- 3. Koshersalt
- 4. Blackpepper
- 5. 20 oz (about 4 cups) cherry tomatoes, halved

METHOD

1. Bring a grill pan or grill grill to medium heat.
2. Slice each squash half in half using a fork. Roast zucchini halves in olive oil and season with salt and pepper on both sides.

3. Put a sizable cast-iron skillet (at least 11") on the grill and heat it for five minutes.
4. Add the olive oil, red onion, cilantro, grated cheese, 3 tablespoons water, and half of the ripped basil.
5. Cook, stirring often, for about 25 minutes or until the tomatoes burst and the mixture becomes aubergine.
6. When the tomatoes are cooking, crush them with a spoon to break them down.
7. Meanwhile, place the chopped zucchini on a grill and cook for approximately 12 minutes on each side or until tender.
8. Once cooked, remove the grill's remaining liquid.
9. Place the grilled zucchini into the tomato sauce and drizzle with olive oil.
10. Place the fresh mozzarella over the top and cover the grill for five minutes to melt the cheese.

11. Serve the grilled zucchini slices on pita bread and top with the leftover shredded basil.
12. Consume right away.

Occasional Egg

Consume no more than three eggs weekly.

Eggs are eaten in all five Blue Zones diets, an average of two to four times weekly. When combined with animal products, eggs make a healthy dish alongside a larger portion of whole grains or other plant-based foods. With a side of beans, Nicoyans fry an egg to roll into a corn tortilla. Boiled eggs are used in Okinawan soups. People in the Mediterranean region fried eggs as a side dish with bread, almonds, and olive oil for breakfast.

Eggs in the Blue Zone diet originate from chickens who roam freely, consume a broad range of naturally occurring foods, do not receive hormones or antibiotics, and lay slowly-matured eggs naturally enriched in omega-3 fatty acids. Eggs produced by hatcheries mature approximately twice as quickly as eggs laid by chickens in blue zones.

Complete proteins, such as amino acids required for your body's B vitamins, vitamins A, D, and E, and minerals like selenium, are all found in eggs. Data from the Adventist Health Study 2 revealed that vegetarians who ate eggs lived marginally longer than non-vegetarians despite their tendency to gain weight.

Other health concerns could impact your decision to include eggs in your Blue Zones diet. Diabetes patients should exercise caution while consuming egg yolks since high egg yolk consumption in males worsens kidney difficulties in women. Despite the ongoing debate among experts over the impact of dietary choices on arterial health, some individuals with cardiovascular or metabolic issues choose not to participate in the debate.

How to go about doing it:

+ Only purchase one little egg from a pastured, cage-free hen.

+ Top a one-egg breakfast with fruit or plant-based foods like bread or wholegrain porridge.

+ Consider substituting scrambled tofu for eggs in your Blue Zones diet.

+ To replace one egg while baking, use a quarter cup of applesauce, a small handful of chopped potatoes, or a tiny banana. Additionally, agar (a substance derived from algae) and flaxseeds can be used in recipes that call for eggs.

6. Daily Amount of Bee Anis

Consume at least one half-cup of cooked beans every day.

The staple of every Blue Zones diet across the globe is beans:

Black beans in Nicoya

Lentils, green beans, and white beans in the Mediterranean

Soybeans in Okinawa

On average, the long-lived populations in these blue zones consume four times as much beansas we do. A five-county study funded by the World Health Organization discovered that eating 20 grams of beans daily decreased a person's risk of dying within a given year by approximately 8%.

The truth is that beans are the most common superfood in the Blue Zone diet. They consist, on average, of 21% protein, 77% complex carbohydrates (the kind that gives you a steady, gradual energy instead of the kind you get from refined carbohydrates, like white flour), and very little fat. They are also a very good source of fiber. They come in various textures, are inexpensive and versatile, and contain more nutrients per gram than any other food on the planet.

Eating beavers has been a part of human culture for at least 8,000 years. Even Daniel's book "Bible" (1:1-21) suggests a two-week vegan diet to improve children's health. A half-cup daily, on average, of blue algae your body needs. Additionally, beans are so hearty and filling that they'll probably force less healthful foods out of your diet. Furthermore, the high fiber content in beans promotes a healthy intestinal flora.

How to go about doing it:

+ Learn how to cook beans as a part of a Blue Zones diet that tastes good to you and your family. The blue zone's centenarians know how to prepare beans to taste excellent. If you don't already have a favorite recipe, consider trying three beaan recipes next month.

Ensure that your kitchen cupboard has a variety of beans available for preparation. While canned beans are pricier, dry beans are more affordable. Make sure you read the label before purchasing canned beans. The only ingredients listed should be beans, water, peppers, and some salt. Steer clear of brands that have added sugar or fat.

+ On the Blue Zone diet, use pureed beans as a thickening to make soups creamy and flavorful.

+ You may make them healthier by adding some cooked beans to them. Serve black bean cakes or hummus alongside salads for a pop of flavor and texture.

+ Always have condiments on hand to spice up and make bean recipes delicious. For instance, Mediterranean bean recipes typically contain carrots, celery, and onions and are spiced with parsley, thyme, pepper, and bay leaves. This is a simple method to incorporate a Blue Zones diet.

+ Consider Mexican restaurants when you dine; they almost always provide pinto or black beans. Improve the bean mixture using red pepper, onion, garlic, and hot sauce. Avoid using white flour tortillas. Rather, choose corn tortillas, which are consumed in Costa Rica.

7. Sugar Scratch

Consume no more than seven tablespoons every day.

Typically, centenarians only eat during festivities. Their diet contains no added sugar, and they usually use honey to sweeten their tea. This adds up to almost seven teaspoons of sugar per day in the diets of the Blue Zones. The lesson to us is:

Savor baked goods, candies, and baked goods only a few times a week, ideally as a meal.

Avoid foods that have added sugar.

Suggest any product where Õugar is one of the first five ingredients mentioned.

Limit the salt added to tea, coffee, or other foods to four tablespoons daily.

Break the habit of munching on sugary, heavy snacks.

Let's face it: Sugar is unavoidable. It naturally occurs in fruits, vegetables, and even milk. However, that is not the issue. Between 1970 and 2000, there was a 25% increase in vegetables added to food. This contributes to the approximately 22 teaspoons of added sugar that the typical American consumes daily—dairy products, including milk, yogurt, eggs, juices, and extra sugars. Excessive sugar intake has been demonstrated to suppress the immune system, making it more difficult to fend off diseases.

Additionally, it lowers insulin levels, which can cause diabetes, impair fertility, make you overweight, and even shorten your life. People on the Blue Zone diet consume around but only around 5% as much added sugar. The key: Individuals in the blue zone consume sugar consciously, not habitually or accidentally.

How to go about doing it:

+ Make honey your go-to sweetener while following a Blue Zones diet. Granted, honey causes blood sugar levels to increase slightly more than sugar, but it's more difficult to spoon in and doesn't dissolve as well in cold liquids.

As a result, you tend to consume it less frequently and more deliberately. Honey is a complete food product. Certain honey, such as IkarĖan honey, has anti-inflammatory, anti-cancer, and antibacterial properties.

Steer clear of sugar-sweetened teas, sodas, and fruit drinks altogether. Sugar-sweetened soda is the main source of added sugars in our diet; in fact, 50% of weight increase in America since 1970 may be attributed to soft drink consumption. A single can of soda pop contains around ten teaspoons of sugar. If you must drink soda, go for diet soda or, better yet, sparkling or sparkling water.

+ Eat strawberries as a celebratory food. Blue zone residents enjoy sweets, although desserts (cakes, cookies, pastries, and dips of all kinds) are nearly always served as a celebratory meal—during village festivals, after a Sunday meal, or as part of a religious holiday. There are frequently special candies for these unique occasions. Limit diets or treatments to one hundred calories. Eat just one meal a day or a few meals.

+ Chill your delicious delight in an at-home Blue Zone diet. Consume fresh fruit instead of juiced fruit. Fresh fruit contains more water and gives you a fuller feeling with fewer calories. The sugar content of dried fruits, including raisins and dates, is significantly lower than that of a typical portion of the fruit while it is fresh.

+ Watch for processed foods with added sugar, specific sugars, salad dressings, and crackers. Many contain a few teaspoons of extra sugar.

+ Look for low-fat products, many sweetened with agarose to compensate for the lack of fat. For example, some low-fat yogurts frequently contain more sugar—ounce for ounce—than regular soda.

+ If your tea or coffee doesn't taste sweet enough, consider using stevia. Naturally, it's not an authentic portion of the Blue Zone diet, but it's very concentrated, making it likely superior to reconstituted parsley.

WHAT Eating in the Zone entails

THE ZONE'S FUNDAMENTAL TENES

Despite what some individuals may believe, the Zone diet has clear and easy principles.

Then, in certain situations, we might argue that it is just common sense.

The well-known 40/30/30 quantitative rule solves the issue of calculating the calories of individual foods.

It is imperative that 40% of the calories we consume come from carbohydrates, 30% from proteins, and 30% from fats.

Simple tables make this possible.

PARTITIONING OUT MEALS

Meals must be spread out across a full day. Specifically, there should be no more than 4/5 hours between a main meal and a snack and no more than 3 hours between a snack and the next meal (not including nights).

Having a snack 30 minutes before bed is best.

This also depends on our schedules, but even if it isn't always feasible, trying to come as close as possible is still helpful.

This is eating before you are truly hungry, which frequently results in overindulging in food and consuming the incorrect kinds of food.

THE FOOD QUALITY

The Zone diet strongly emphasizes dietary quality.

Thus, it is especially advised to utilize wholegrain grasses as a secondary source of carbs and to use fruits and vegetables as the primary source.

Utilizing mono and polyunsaturated fats—found in olive oil, dried fruit, and the fat of some fish, such as oily fish—is advised by the Zone diet.

Since the Omega 3 series fats are so important, special attention is paid to them.

Lean proteins are desired, focusing on fish and white meat in particular. Vegetable proteins, like those found in legumes, should never be completely absent.

Thus, in general, the Zone diet aligns with the Mediterranean diet, which I discuss right after, at least regarding food quality.

Day Four

• For breakfast, have a two-egg omelet with two slices of whole wheat toast, half a cup of diced tomatoes, and bell peppers.

• Snack: half a cup of blueberries and half a cup of reduced-fat cottage cheese.

- Three ounces of grilled turkey, half a cup of cooked barley, and a cup of steamed broccoli will be served for lunch.
- Snack is a quarter cup of almonds and one piece of fruit.
- Four ounces of roasted beef, twelve cups of bell peppers, and steamed green beans will make up dinner.

Day Five

- One serving of a smoothie for breakfast, consisting of half a cup of nonfat milk, banana, and 1/4 cup of oats.
- A snack of one cup of sliced veggies and half a cup of hummus.
- We'll have half a cup of cooked millet, one cup of steaming greens, and four ounces of grilled chicken for lunch.
- Snack: a quarter cup of granola and a half cup of plain Greek yogurt

- We'll have roasted sweet potatoes, half a cup of cooked quinoa, one cup of asparagus, and four ounces of shrimp for dinner.

Day Six

- We had half a cup of nonfat milk, a quarter cup of walnuts, and a cup of oats for breakfast.
- Snack: one hard-boiled egg and a slice of fruit
- One-fourth of a cup of trail mix as a snack: three ounces of grilled steak with steamed spinach and half a cup of boiled lentils for lunch.
- The meal will be four ounces of roasted pork, one cup of steaming green beans, half a cup of cooked brown rice, and half a cup of roasted bell peppers.

Customizing the Zone diet to meet personal needs

One of the most important ways to ensure the Zone Diet is sustainable, successful, and fits each person's particular needs is to customize it to suit individual needs. The Zone Diet can be tailored by following these steps:

Calorie Needs Calculation: This method calculates your daily energy requirements based on age, height, weight, degree of physical activity, and specific objectives (muscle gain, weight loss, or maintenance).

Establishing the 40-30-30 Ratio: Modify the ratio to your unique requirements and inclinations. Sometimes, making small adjustments to the conventional ratio—for instance, raising the proportion of protein or carbohydrates by a small amount—can be beneficial. Modifying the Block Count:

The daily allotment of blocks may differ. You can change the quantity of blocks depending on your dietary preferences, needs, and calorie requirements.

Food Selection and Nutritious Sources: Select meals that meet your tastes and adhere to the 40-30-30 ratio. Following a diet over time may be simpler if there is flexibility and variety in food options.

Individual Response Monitoring: Pay close attention to how the diet affects your body. Monitor your energy levels, post-meal contentment, physical fitness, and weight control. These elements may affect the required modifications.

Personalizing Proportions: You might discover that a different distribution of macronutrients suits you the best. Adjust the proportions of proteins, carbs, and fats to suit your goals and sense of well-being.

Consultation with a Health expert: You should always get advice from a health expert or dietitian before making big dietary adjustments. They can give you individualized advice and thoroughly study your unique demands.

The key objective is customizing the Zone Diet to your unique goals, food preferences, and lifestyle. Flexibility and personalization are essential for any long-term diet to be successful and sustainable.

Section Three

The Blue Zone Diet Program's advantages

Extended Lifespan

The longer lifetime of humans is one of the biggest advantages of medical science and technology advances. Over the past few decades, life expectancy has increased, and this trend will probably continue in the years to come. The longer lifespan has several effects on people and society at large.

People are more likely to experience chronic illnesses, including diabetes, heart disease, and cancer, as they get older. But because of developments in medicine, people can now live longer and take better care of their chronic illnesses. New therapies and drugs, for example, can help diabetics control their blood sugar levels and lower their risk of problems.

Given that older persons are more likely to need medical attention and social support, this trend substantially impacts social services and healthcare systems. Governments and healthcare organizations must, therefore, invest in new services, technologies, and policies that specifically address the demands of the aging population to meet their evolving needs.

Longer lifespans have an impact on people's and society's finances. Longer lifespans allow people to labor and support the economy for longer, boosting productivity and economic growth. Furthermore, healthy and energetic older persons can engage in social and cultural activities that support a dynamic and diverse community.

It's crucial to remember that living a longer life is difficult. Longer lifespans may increase a person's need for medical attention and social assistance, which could overburden social services and healthcare systems. Furthermore, ageism, discrimination based on age, and social isolation may provide new difficulties for older persons, all of which might lower their quality of life.

Extended life expectancy is a noteworthy accomplishment of contemporary medical science and technology, bearing substantial consequences for individuals and the community. There are chances for innovation and growth in addition to the issues of an aging population.

Reduced Chance of Persistent Illnesses

Globally, chronic illnesses like diabetes and cancer. On the other hand, new therapies for diseases have been made possible by advancements in medical science and technology. These actions have significant effects on both personal and societal health.

Chronic illness risk can be decreased by maintaining a nutritious diet, engaging in regular exercise, abstaining from tobacco use, and limiting alcohol intake. Early chronic disease detection and treatment can also reduce problems and enhance results. For example, routine cancer screenings can identify the illness early on, when it is easier to treat.

Additionally, there are new drugs and therapies available to reduce the risk of chronic illnesses. Statins, for instance, are medications that help lower. Similarly, fresh immunotherapies that target cancer cells and strengthen the immune system are being developed. For those with chronic illnesses, these therapies.

Vaccinations and other preventative measures can help reduce the chance of chronic illnesses. For example, immunizations against the flu can avoid problems in those with chronic diseases, and vaccinations against the human papillomavirus (HPV) can prevent cervical cancer.

Reducing the likelihood of chronic illnesses significantly affects both personal and societal health. Chronic illnesses can have a major negative influence on a person's quality of life and are frequently costly to treat. People can live healthier, more productive lives and benefit society if the risk of certain diseases is reduced.

Still, there are difficulties in both treating and preventing chronic illnesses. For example, certain societies may restrict access to healthcare and preventative measures, disproportionately affecting underprivileged populations. Furthermore, there is still a great deal to learn about the etiology and risk factors of chronic illnesses, which can complicate prevention and therapy.

Despite these difficulties, one important development in modern medicine and technology is the growing availability of medicines, lifestyle modifications, and preventative measures to reduce the risk of chronic diseases. Healthcare systems can keep improving the lives of those with chronic illnesses and keep these illnesses from posing a serious threat to the public's health by funding research and development.

Why Are Salads Used?

Typically, lettuce serves as the foundation of a salad because it is high in fiber and packed with nutrients. Because lettuce contains vitamins C, E, and K—essential for developing collagen and elastin—greens are excellent for skin, hair, and digestive health, as well as detoxifying and purifying the body. The best food for anti-aging is lettuce. Fiber is essential to maintain a sensation of fullness and satisfaction. One of the best foods for summer is a salad. Put some nuts or seeds in your salads to replace the high-carb croutons. You can replace croutons with nuts or seeds because most croutons aren't prepared with entire grains. Eating seeds is a simple approach to increasing nutrient intake while consuming fewer calories from simple carbohydrates.

● For that crunch factor salad topper you've been craving without the bad carbs, try adding some protein to your dish with raw nuts like pecans, almonds, walnuts, and pepitas. Regarding salad dressings, steer clear of store-bought varieties, as most are high in fattening preservatives.

● Make your salad dressings; this is a simple tip.

Simply drizzle your homemade dressing over your salad and enjoy! To make your own, combine one tablespoon of plain yogurt with your preferred seed oil, such as olive or hemp oil, herbs, red wine vinegar, balsamic vinegar, or freshly squeezed orange or lemon juice.

More Antioxidants Are Found in Lettuce Than in Salmon Omega

Choose foods strong in antioxidants and Omega 3, 6, and 9 content, such as salmon, eggs, and lettuce. Omegas maintain healthy skin, strong nails, and glossy hair. Consume abundant fruits and nuts, such as walnuts and almonds; red fruits and vegetables, such as pomegranates, grapes, tomatoes, and strawberries, are the best. Consume raw vegetables like bell peppers, carrots, and blueberries regularly. Consuming meals high in collagen and protein will keep your body strong, and including them in your beauty routine can also greatly benefit it. Using foods like a range of lettuces, the v-Diet is a therapeutic approach to provide your family with greater health, energy, enhanced beauty, and longevity. Maintaining your health as you age largely depends on eating a well-balanced diet. It can support you in getting the nutrients you require, staying energized, and maintaining a healthy weight. It also lessens your chance of getting long-term illnesses like diabetes and heart disease. Food and beverages serve as more than just our bodies' nourishment. Food is more than physical sustenance; it fosters positive relationships and family or group bonding moments. After work, families use dinner to catch up, have one-on-one conversations, and share stories from the day. Mealtimes should be stress-free occasions to unwind and enjoy mindful eating.

Types of Raw Vegetables and Lettuces That Can Replace Crackers Try substituting crunchy vegetables for toast and crackers in your diet to get rid of processed wheat and grain carbohydrates.

● Endive Lettuce: Endive gives a substantial crunch to lettuce.

● Sweet potato sticks are crunchy and sweet;
● Carrot sticks are crunchy and sweet; ● Celery sticks are crunchy and salty; ● Little

Gem lettuce is soft with a hint of crunch; ● Romaine lettuce is crisp and robust;

Cucumber Slices: crispy and succulent

Consume Crispy Lettuce Rather Than Crackers

Eating crunchy vegetables with dips, hummus, cheese, and nut butter is a healthy way to substitute crackers if you're trying to cut out processed wheat and grain carbohydrates from your diet.

An alternative to crackers

Other Crunchy Veggie Options To Replace Crackers and Toast: ● Sushi wrap seaweed paper ● Romaine Lettuce – a long leaf that is crunchy and hearty ● Little Gem Lettuce – soft with just a hint of crunch ● Belgian Endive Lettuce Leaves – endive adds a solid crunch ● Crisp plantain; crunchy and sweet carrot sticks; crunchy and salty celery sticks

■ Crunchy and delicious sweet potato sticks ■ Crunchy radish slices

- Crunchy and moist cucumber slices

Substitutes for Crackers:

Traditional wheat flour-based crackers are heavy in lipids, calories, and carbohydrates. Many individuals choose to make vegetable chips from dehydrated kale or spinach since they are a healthier alternative to fried variety flavor potato chips or white flour crackers.

Japanese Miso Soup: Savoury Drink For Extended Lifespan

Ingredients:

- 2 green onions, thinly sliced
- 1 cup sliced mushrooms (shiitake or button)
- 1 tablespoon soy sauce (optional)
- Sliced radishes for garnish (optional)
- 4 cups water
- 2 tablespoons miso paste (white or red)
- 1 cup tofu, cubed
- 1 cup seaweed (wakame), rehydrated and chopped

Instructions:

1. Four cups of water should be brought to a medium simmer in a saucepan.

2. Use a few tablespoons of hot water. This keeps it from clumping together when you add it to the soup.
3. Add the tofu, seaweed, mushrooms, and green onions to the simmering water.
4. Sauté the mushrooms for five to seven minutes or until they are soft.
5. After adding the dissolved miso paste, boil the soup for two to three minutes.
6. Miso can become gritty if boiled, so don't do so.
7. If you want more flavor, taste the soup and add soy sauce if you so like.
8. Spoon the miso soup into individual bowls, and feel free to top with sliced radishes.
9. Serve hot for a calming, umami-rich beverage.

Blue Zone Dietary Guidelines

An Extensive Inventory of Foods Typically Found in Blue Zone Areas

Some areas of the world are known as "blue zones," where people typically live longer and in better health. These cultures' distinct diets have been linked, among other things, to their lifespan and general wellbeing. This section will discuss the typical foods found in Blue Zone areas and how they support the citizens' overall health and wellbeing.

1. Green leafy vegetables

Diets in the Blue Zone are heavy in leafy greens. Vitamins A, C, and K, fiber, and folate are just a few vital elements in varieties like kale, spinach, and collard greens. These greens are essential to a balanced diet because they are high in nutrients and low in calories.

2. Legumes & Beans

Legumes and beans, like black beans, chickpeas, and lentils, are high in fiber, complex carbs, and plant-based protein. They lower the chance of overeating by supplying steady energy, assisting with blood sugar regulation, and promoting a feeling of fullness.

3. Complete Grains

Whole grains, such as quinoa and barley, are consumed by people living in the Blue Zone. Whole grains help digestion, heart health, and sustained daily energy levels.

4. Seeds and Nuts

Among the nuts and seeds common in Blue Zone diets are almonds, walnuts, and flaxseeds. They provide protein, various vitamins and minerals, and healthy fats. In addition to sating hunger, these snacks.

5. Fruits: Fruits like oranges, apples, and blueberries are plentiful in the Blue Zone. Antioxidants, vitamins, and dietary fiber—all critical for maintaining general health and preventing disease—are abundant in these fruits.

6. Fish Fish is a staple food in coastal Blue Zone locations. Omega-3 fatty acids are found in fish, especially fatty types like mackerel and salmon,

7. Extra Virgin Olive Oil

A key component of Blue Zone cooking is olive oil. It has a lot of monounsaturated fats, which are good for the heart, and antioxidants, which fight oxidative stress. Olive oil is a common healthy salad dressing and cooking oil.

8. Spices and Herbs

Spices and herbs give Blue Zone cuisine depth and taste without using a lot of salt or bad fats. Herbs like basil, rosemary, and oregano are often utilized, and spices like cinnamon and turmeric have several health advantages.

9. Water Blue Zone people usually drink a lot of water during the day because it's important for their health to stay properly hydrated. Maintaining adequate hydration promotes healthy circulation, digestion, and general energy.

10. Red wine (sans added sugar)

Red wine is consumed in moderation in several Blue Zone villages. Resveratrol, an antioxidant found in red wine, may support heart health. To get the potential advantages without the hazards, alcohol must be consumed in moderation.

Including these foods in your diet derived from Blue Zone areas can help you live longer and be healthier. They greatly complement anyone's eating habits because of their plant-based, high-nutrient content, which aligns with the concepts of balanced nutrition.

Bread made with Sardinia whole grains and olive oil

Ingredients: - Whole grain bread (you may use any kind of whole grain bread) - Extra virgin olive oil

- Optional sea salt

Guidelines:

1. Choose the Bread: If you can, start with a high-quality Sardinian wholegrain bread. It's a healthier option because wholegrain bread is high in minerals and fiber. But feel free to use any kind of wholegrain bread you like.

2. Cut the Bread: Cut the bread into thick, rustic slices using a sharp knife. Though a substantial thickness is advised, you can create them as thin or thick as you desire.

3. Toast the Bread: Depending on your tastes. The bread will stay naturally soft if it is not toasted, but it will have a lovely crunch if it is.

4. Drizzle with Olive Oil: Arrange the bread pieces on a tray or separate plates. Spread a liberal amount of extra virgin olive oil on the bread. Don't be afraid to use plenty of olive oil in this recipe; its rich, fruity flavor is essential.

5. Optional Sea Salt Sprinkle: You may want to top the olive oil with a small pinch of sea salt.

This gives a mild, savory note that balances the richness of the olive oil.

6. Serve: Now is the time to present your Sardinian Whole Grain Bread with Olive Oil. This light and tasty recipe let the natural flavors of the bread and olive oil shine through. Savor it as an appetizer, a snack, or with other dishes that have a Mediterranean influence.

The Function of Communities and Lifestyle Zones Due to Regional and Cultural Disparities. Nonetheless, the following diet is primarily plant- and whole-food-based, characterized by moderation, mindful eating, and social interaction. These dietary guidelines align with increasing research demonstrating improved longevity and well-being.

Comprehending the significance of community and lifestyle is essential to appreciate the longevity and well-being observed in Blue Zones, where people frequently have exceptionally long and prosperous lives. These communities have shared lifestyle traits that greatly enhance the wellbeing and longevity of their members. An examination of the significance of community and lifestyle in Blue Zones is provided here:

1. Sturdy Social Networks: Strong social ties significantly impact Blue Zones. Residents frequently uphold close-knit communities where routine interactions with family, friends, and neighbors are the norm. These social ties foster a sense of purpose and belonging, lessen stress, and provide emotional support.

2. Feeling of Identity: Blue Zone residents have a strong sense of community inside their neighborhoods. This sense of being a complete social network member promotes emotional health and lessens feelings of loneliness or isolation.

3. Community Meals: In Blue Zones, meals are typically shared with the community. Friends and family get together to share laughs, stories,

and cuisine. These shared meal experiences foster a sense of community and strengthen bonds between people.

4. Physical Activity Integrated: In Blue Zones, physical activity is a seamless part of everyday life. Instead of structured workouts, people engage in natural exercise like walking, gardening, or manual labor. A lifestyle this active promotes overall health and vigor.

5. Practices for Stress Management: Residents of Blue Zones frequently include stress management techniques into their everyday routines, whether through consistent social interactions, mindfulness exercises, or relaxation techniques. A lower risk of chronic illnesses has been associated with lower stress levels.

6. Living Purposefully: A prominent feature in Blue Zones is a strong sense of meaning and purpose in life. Residents participate in activities that give them a cause to get out of

bed in the morning, such as taking care of their gardens, attending community events, or following personal interests.

7. Respect for Elderly Members: Blue Zone communities frequently strongly regard their elderly members. Elderly people are respected for their knowledge and experience and still actively participate in their communities.

8. Complementary Environments: Blue Zones are intended to encourage affluent life. Residents' wellbeing is influenced by various factors, including walkableneighborhoods, access to fresh, locally sourced food, and environments that promote physical exercise.

9. Cultural customs: Many Blue Zone communities have customs and traditions that bolster social ties and overall wellbeing. These customs frequently centeraround storytelling, dancing, and food.

10. Lifelong Education: Throughout their lives, residents of Blue Zones frequently engage in

learning. Constant mental stimulation and curiosity support mental wellbeing and a sense of direction.

11. Shared values: Blue Zone communities frequently share values such as respect for nature, an emphasis on family, and a dedication to health and wellbeing. These common values promoted a sense of cohesion and solidarity.

Blue Zones' emphasis on lifestyle and community underscores. These elements create a supportive environment where people make decisions that enhance their health and longevity. People in other regions can improve their quality of life, encourage better health, and potentially extend their years of wellbeing by adopting elements of the Blue Zone lifestyle.

Chapter 3: Using the Zone Diet to Supplement Your Training Program

You now know a lot about the foods you should be consuming, so it's time to concentrate on planning your daily meals according to the type of training you are doing and the time of day. I'll share the expertise I've gained over my last ten years as a professional cross-trainer. The 40:30:30 rule, zone blocking, figuring out the best zone blocking for each meal, and how NOT to break the zone diet plan every time you eat out will be covered here.

The 40:30:30 rule's fundamentals

The 40:30:30 guideline counters the most important component of the Zone Diet plan. As was previously mentioned, the human body needs to be fed 40% carbohydrates, 30% protein, and 30% fat daily to maintain optimal health and promote quick muscle building and fat reduction. As Sears puts it, "staying in the zone"—a term he likes to use—is made possible by a balanced diet. Hormones regulate insulin, glucagon, and eicosanoids, which propels us to perform throughout the day. This has been demonstrated beyond a shadow of a doubt.

What roles do these hormones play? Insulin, on the other hand, is a hormone that helps you store fat; glucagon, on the other hand, is a hormone that mobilizes stored carbohydrates; and eicosanoids, on the other hand, are the main hormones that govern the activity of other hormones in our body. It should go without saying that producing too much of any one of these three hormones can have fatal consequences. This is precisely what the Zone Diet aids in controlling.

The zone block and its measurement

The Zone Diet is measured in blocks, and the best way to attain hormonal balance and total mental and physical wellbeing is to plan meals based on the Zone block charts. This diet guarantees you all the nutrients you need to stay at the top of your game all day, regardless of whether you are a professional athlete looking to switch to the Zone Diet or someone just starting with cross-training.

You must account for your body type and size when calculating the block required. I have the appropriate kinds of Zone blocks available for you, regardless of how big, small, or in between they are. As a nutritionist and fitness specialist, I suppose that choosing the right diet plan may appear complex initially. But hang on! Everything you need to know about zone blocking will be made simple for you by me.

Veggie Breakfast Burritos

Ingredients:

- 1/2 cup black beans, drained and rinsed
- 1/2 cup shredded cheese (optional)
- Salt and pepper to taste
- 4 large tortillas (whole grain or gluten-free, as desired)
- 6 large eggs, scrambled

- 1 cup mixed vegetables (such as bell peppers, onions, and zucchini), diced
- Salsa, avocado, or sour cream for serving (optional)

Instructions:

1. Heat the mixed veggies in the quick electric pressure cooker using the "Saute" setting until they soften.
2. Cook the black beans and scrambled eggs in the cooker until the beans are heated and thoroughly cooked.
3. Add pepper and salt for seasoning.
4. Move the veggie and egg mixture to one side of the cooker so that there is room for the tortillas to warm up.
5. Using tongs, flip each tortilla and place it directly on the bottom of the cooker for a

few seconds on each side or until it is heated.
6. Place a spoonful of the egg and veggie mixture onto each tortilla, and if you like, top it with shredded cheese.
7. Enclose the filling by rolling the tortillas and tucking in the edges.
8. top the breakfast burritos with sour cream, avocado, or salsa if preferred.

Cooking Tip: Tailor the burrito fillings to your tastes. For additional taste, you can also add herbs or spices.

Nutritional Information: These breakfast burritos contain a ton of veggies, protein, and good fats.

Why Blue Zone Smoothies in Chapter 3?

Smoothies—those amazing concoctions of fruit and other ingredients that have been around for decades—have grown in popularity as a quick and healthful beverage choice for health-conscious people. However, not every smoothie is created equal. How do you tell which products are healthy when so many are on the market? Let us introduce Blue Zone Smoothies.

Only the freshest, natural ingredients, grown and harvested at the peak of their flavor and nutritional value, go into making Blue Zone Smoothies. They are abundant in vital components needed for. Blue Zone Smoothies are made without artificial sweeteners, preservatives, or additional sugars, so you know you're getting the real deal.

Blue Zone Smoothies' special ingredient balance is their key to success. The main component, blueberries, provides each smoothie with flavor and nutrition. Antioxidant-rich blueberries help reduce inflammation and provide a natural energy boost. Crucial vitamins and minerals in blueberries include magnesium, potassium, and vitamin C, all essential for overall health and well-being.

Almond milk, bananas, pineapple, and coconut are added ingredients in Blue Zone Smoothies. Pineapple offers a tropical flavor and a good amount of vitamin C, while bananas offer a natural sweetness and a fantastic source of potassium.

Almond and coconut milk are excellent for adding a creamy texture to smoothies and are also great sources of good fats.

Blue Zone Smoothies are a convenient and nutritious way to get your recommended daily intake of nutrients while on the go. These smoothies could be a satisfying and healthful snack for you in the middle of the afternoon or as a quick breakfast. And making them couldn't be easier: just combine all the ingredients in a blender, and you're set to go.

So look no further than Blue Zone Smoothies for a well-balanced, nutrient-dense snack or meal replacement. Their special blend of natural ingredients offers a great way to get a cute, practical bottle. So, try a Blue Zone Smoothie for your next meal or snack instead of reaching for sugar-filled drinks and snacks. You won't be sorry!

Greek Salad

Ingredients:

- 1/2 cup Kalamata olives
- 1/2 cup crumbled feta cheese
- 2 tablespoons extra-virgin olive oil
- 1 tablespoon lemon juice
- **2 cups mixed salad greens**
- 1 cucumber, diced
- 1 cup cherry tomatoes, halved
- 1/2 red onion, thinly sliced
- 1 teaspoon dried oregano
- Salt and pepper to taste

Instructions:

1. Feta cheese in a big salad dish.
2. Mix the olive oil, lemon juice, dried oregano, salt, and pepper in a small bowl.
3. After drizzling the salad with the dressing, gently toss to coat.
4. Serve right away.

Oatmeal with Blueberries

Ingredients:

- 1 cup blueberries (fresh or frozen)
- 1 tablespoon maple syrup (optional)
- 1 teaspoon vanilla extract
- 1 cup steel-cut oats
- 2 cups water
- 1 cup almond milk

Instructions:

1. Combine all ingredients in the electric pressure cooker.
2. After four minutes of high-pressure cooking, close the cover.
3. After the cooking time is over, execute a fast release after letting the pressure release normally for ten minutes.
4. Before serving, give the oats a good stir.
5. top with more ingredients like honey drizzled over or sliced almonds if desired.

Cooking Tip: To ensure the blueberries are distributed equally, thoroughly stir the oatmeal before serving. Add extra almond milk if you'd like the texture to be creamier.

Nutritional Information: Plant-based protein, fiber, and antioxidants are abundant in this recipe.

Apple Cinnamon Quinoa

Ingredients:

- 1 tablespoon maple syrup (optional)
- 1 teaspoon ground cinnamon
- 1/4 teaspoon ground nutmeg (optional)
- 1 cup quinoa, rinsed
- 1 cup water
- 1 cup almond milk
- 1 apple, peeled, cored, and diced

Instructions:

1. Add the quinoa, water, almond milk, diced apple, maple syrup, cinnamon, and nutmeg to the quick electric pressure cooker.
2. After eight minutes of high-pressure cooking, close the cover.
3. After the cooking time is over, execute a fast release after letting the pressure release generally for ten minutes.
4. Using a fork, fluff the quinoa and serve it warm.
5. If preferred, sprinkle with chopped nuts or raisins, or use more almond milk.

Recipes For Blue Zone Green Smoothies

Ingredients:

- -1/2 cup almond milk
- -½ teaspoon powdered ginger
- -1/2 teaspoon crushed turmeric

- -1 banana
- -1 cup blueberries
- -1 cup spinach
- -1 tablespoon honey

Instructions:

1. Blend the banana, almond milk, spinach, blueberries, ginger, turmeric, and honey until smooth.
2. Serve right away.

www.ingramcontent.com/pod-product-compliance
Lightning Source LLC
Chambersburg PA
CBHW070031040426
42333CB00040B/1531